ESSENTIAL ACTINIC KERATOSIS

Comprehensive Diagnosis, Treatment, and Prevention Strategies for Dermatological Health

DR. CASEY LOREN

© 2024 by CASEY LOREN

All rights reserved .Except for brief quotations included in critical reviews and certain other noncommercial uses allowed by copyright law, no part of this book may be reproduced, distributed, or transmitted in any form or by any means, including photocopying, recording, or other electronic or mechanical methods, without the publisher's prior written permission.

DISCLAIMER

This book's content is only meant to be used for general informative purposes. Although the author has taken great care to ensure the content is accurate and thorough, no warranties or assurances on the information's accuracy, correctness, or reliability are provided. It is recommended that readers employ their own judgment and discretion when applying any material found in this book to their particular situation.

The information in this book is not intended to replace professional advice, nor is the author an expert in any of the subjects covered. It is recommended that readers consult with experienced professionals regarding any particular issues or concerns.

Any name that may be mentioned or referred in this book does not imply endorsement, recommendation, or relationship on the part of the author with any person, entity, good, website, or association. These references are made only for informational purposes and are not meant to be taken as recommendations or endorsements.

The information contained in this book may cause readers to suffer loss or damage, for which the author disclaims all obligation and accountability. The only people accountable for the decisions and actions taken by readers using the information presented are themselves.

Any names, characters, companies, locations, activities, occasions, and incidents referenced in this book are either made up or the result of the author's imagination. Any likeness to real people, living or dead, or to real things is entirely coincidental.

This book's content may change at any time, without prior notice, according to the author.

The onus is on the reader to verify whether there have been any updates or revisions.

The reader accepts the conditions of this disclaimer by reading this book. Please do not read this book or use its contents if you do not agree to these terms.

Table of Contents

CHAPTER 1 16

OVERVIEW OF ACTINIC KERATOSIS 16

Comprehensive Handbook on Actinic Keratosis 16

Actinic Keratosis: Definition and Synopsis 16

Prevalence and Epidemiology 17

Risk Factors for Actinic Keratosis Development 17

- **Age**: 18

- **complexion Type**: 18

- **History of Sunburns**: 18

- **Immunosuppression**: 18

- **Genetic Factors**: 18

Actinic Keratosis Pathogenesis 19

Symptoms and Clinical Presentation 19

Tools and Techniques for Diagnostics 20

Significance of Prompt Identification 21

Effect on Life Quality 21

Available Treatments Right Now 22

   - **Cryotherapy**: 22

   - **Photodynamic Therapy (PDT)**: 23

   - **Chemical Peels**: 23

   - **Laser Therapy**: 23

   - **Surgical Removal**: 23

Prospects for Further Actinic Keratosis Research 24

   Advanced Imaging Techniques: 24

   - **Immunotherapy**: 24

   Gene Therapy: 25

   Preventive Strategies: 25

CHAPTER 2 26

RECOGNIZING UV RADIATION AND SUN DAMAGE 26

UV Radiation's Effects on Skin 26

   - **DNA Damage**: 26

- **Inflammation**: 27

- **Immunological Suppression**: 27

- **Protein Damage**: 27

The Distinction Between UVA and UVB Radiation 27

The UVA (320–400 nm) rays: 28

- **UVB Rays: 290–320 nanometers): 28

Photoaging and Skin Ageing 29

Actinic Keratosis and UV Exposure Relationship 30

Sun Protection Is Crucial 31

Frequently Held Myths Regarding Sunscreen 32

UV Index and Hazard Evaluation 33

Strategies for Photoprotection 34

Including Sun-Safe Practices in Everyday Activities 35

UV Protection Public Health Initiatives 35

CHAPTER 3 38

RISK ELEMENTS AND PREVENTIVE TECHNIQUES 38

Genetic Predisposition and Skin Type 38

Causes of Actinic Keratosis in the Environment..39

Workplace Risks and Sun Exposure 39

Living Decisions and Their Effects 40

Immune Suppression's Role 40

Prevention via Early Childhood Education ..41

Programmes for Community-Based Prevention..42

CHAPTER 4..44

CLINICAL ASSESSMENT AND IDENTIFICATION 44

Significance of Skin Exams 44

Crucial Elements for Recognising Actinic Keratosis Lesions..45

Differential Diagnoses and Related Illnesses 46

Histopathological Examination and Biopsy Methods 47

Actinic Keratosis Diagnosis Using Dermoscopy 49

Photography's Function in Tracking Injuries 50

Remote Diagnosis and Teledermatology 51

Educating Patients During the Diagnosis 52

Diagnosis's Psychological Impact 53

Using a Multidisciplinary Method to Diagnose 54

CHAPTER 5 58

   METHODS OF TREATMENT 58

   Actinic Keratosis Topical Treatments 58

   Surgical Removal and Resection 64

   Chemical Peels for the Treatment of Actinic Keratosis 66

   Agents Immunomodulatory 67

Combination Treatments for Immune Toxins 69

Post-treatment patient monitoring and follow-up 71

CHAPTER 6 74

HANDLING ACTINIC KERATOSIS IN PARTICULAR GROUPS 74

Pediatric Patients with Actinic Keratosis: 74

Geriatric Issues and Difficulties: 75

In Immunocompromised Individuals: Actinic Keratosis 76

Managing Actinic Keratosis During Pregnancy: 76

Differences in Presentation by Culture and Ethnicity: 77

Access to Care and Socioeconomic Factors: 78

Patient Psychological Support: 78

Approaches in Integrated Medicine: 79

Advanced Cases: Palliative Care 79

Family and Carer Support: 81

CHAPTER 7 82

ISSUES AND PROLONGED CONSEQUENCES 82

Squamous Cell Carcinoma Progression 83

Advanced Lesions' Metastatic Potential 83

Rates of Recurrence Following Treatment .. 84

Cosmetic Concerns and Scar Formation 85

Functional Deficit Owing to Injuries 85

Effect of Psychology on Life Quality 86

Monitoring Techniques for Patients at High Risk 87

Supplementary Preventive Actions 87

Long-Term Results Research 88

Attending to Patient Worries Regarding Complications 89

CHAPTER 8 92

Instruction for Patients and Self-Management 92

Patient Education Is Critical for Actinic Keratosis 92

Comprehending the Objectives and Treatment Options 93

Methods for Self-Examination 94

Sun Safety Procedures for Everyday Living . 95

Changes in Lifestyle to Prevent 96

Tracking and Reporting Modifications to Lesions 97

Following Treatment Plans 98

Patient Support Resources 99

Providing Knowledge To Empower Patients 100

Formulating Customised Treatment Programmes 101

CHAPTER NINE.. 104

POLICY ASPECTS OF PUBLIC IIEALTII .. 104

Actinic Keratosis's Cost to Healthcare Systems 104

Incidence and Prevalence: 105

Medical Service Usage: 105

Actinic Keratosis's Economic Impact..........106

Health Policies to Prevent Skin Cancer......108

The Function of NGOs and the Government in Awareness Campaigns 110

Insurance Protection for the Management of Actinic Keratosis..113

Priorities and Funding for Research 115

Promoting the Avoidance of Skin Cancer ...116

CHAPTER 10 120

   UPCOMING DEVELOPMENTS AND TRENDS..120

   Technological Developments in Actinic Keratosis Detection.......................................120

   Personalised medicine and targeted therapies 122

   Development of Vaccines and Immunotherapy 123

Treatment Applications of Nanotechnology 124

Dermatology and Artificial Intelligence 126

Digital health and telemedicine solutions ..127

Comprehensive Methods for Skin Health ..128

Innovations Focused on the Patient 129

Redefining Actinic Keratosis Treatment in the Future 131

CHAPTER 1

OVERVIEW OF ACTINIC KERATOSIS

Comprehensive Handbook on Actinic Keratosis

Actinic Keratosis: Definition and Synopsis

Actinic Keratosis (AK), sometimes referred to as solar keratosis, is a common skin ailment that appears as scaly, rough patches on skin that have been exposed to sunlight. Long-term cumulative exposure to ultraviolet (UV) radiation, mostly from the sun, causes these lesions. Because they may develop into squamous cell carcinoma (SCC), a kind of skin cancer, AKs are regarded as precancerous. Even obviously not all AK will develop into cancer, their existence suggests severe sun damage and a higher risk of skin cancer.

Prevalence and Epidemiology

Actinic Keratosis is common throughout the world, particularly in areas with intense sun exposure. Fair-skinned people are most affected since they are more vulnerable to UV damage. Research indicates that the frequency rises with age, with over 50% of adults over 50 in areas with significant UV exposure having at least one AK lesion. One of the most prevalent dermatological disorders in the US, AKs are thought to affect about 58 million people.

Risk Factors for Actinic Keratosis Development

Long-term exposure to UV radiation from the sun or tanning beds is the main risk factor for AK. Other risk variables consist of:

- **Age**: The cumulative effect of solar exposure over time puts older people at increased risk.

- **complexion Type**: Blond or red hair, light-colored eyes, and fair complexion all increase the risk of AKs.

- **Geographic Location**: UV exposure is higher in areas with lots of sunshine or at high elevations.

- **History of Sunburns**: The risk is increased by severe or frequent sunburns, particularly in infancy.

- **Immunosuppression**: AKs are more common among people with compromised immune systems, such as organ transplant recipients.

- **Genetic Factors**: Some genetic profiles may make a person more vulnerable to UV rays.

Actinic Keratosis Pathogenesis

UV light damages DNA, which results in mutations in the keratinocytes—the main epidermal cells—and causes actinic keratosis. The damage causes aberrant cell division and proliferation, which gives rise to dysplastic, precancerous lesions. Additionally, UV light inhibits the skin's local immune responses, which permits the survival and growth of these aberrant cells.

Symptoms and Clinical Presentation

Small, rough, scaly patches on sun-exposed areas including the face, ears, neck, scalp, shoulders, and hands are the characteristic appearance of AK lesions. They can appear skin-toned, pink, red, or brown, depending on their color. AKs are frequently compared to sandpaper in texture. Although lesions are normally asymptomatic, they might burn, itch, or feel sensitive. It is typical for several lesions to combine to form bigger, more pronounced patches.

Tools and Techniques for Diagnostics

Actinic keratosis is mostly diagnosed clinically, using the patient's medical history and characteristic appearance as guidelines. Dermatologists can see the lesions more clearly by using dermoscopy, a non-invasive device that magnifies the skin. In cases of uncertainty, a skin biopsy could be necessary to distinguish AK from other illnesses such as basal cell carcinoma (BCC) or SCC. The diagnosis is confirmed by histological analysis of the biopsy sample, which shows atypical keratinocytes restricted to the lower epidermis.

Significance of Prompt Identification

Early identification of AK is essential for timely treatment, which lowers the chance that the condition will advance to SCC. A dermatologist's routine skin inspections, especially for high-risk patients, can detect lesions early on when they are easier to cure. Additionally, early intervention enhances the long-term health of the skin and helps control the overall burden of UV damage.

Effect on Life Quality

The quality of life can be greatly affected by actinic keratosis, particularly if there are many lesions or if they are noticeable and appear on the hands and face. The anxiety associated with the possibility of cancer spreading and the aesthetic worries can hurt an individual's mental health and self-worth. The uncomfortable and negative effects of the treatment methods, which could include cryotherapy, topical drugs, or photodynamic therapy, further interfere with day-to-day functioning.

Available Treatments Right Now

The goals of treating AK include symptom relief, stopping the spread of the disease to SCC, and removing or destroying the precancerous cells. Typical therapies consist of:

- **Cryotherapy**: Use liquid nitrogen to freeze the lesion, causing it to blister and fall off.

- **Topical Medications**: Creams or gels that encourage the elimination of aberrant cells, such as imiquimod, diclofenac, and 5-fluorouracil.

- **Photodynamic Therapy (PDT)**: Using a photosensitizing chemical and a particular light wavelength, aberrant cells are destroyed.

- **Chemical Peels**: Chemical solutions are applied to the skin to remove layers of damage.

- **Laser Therapy**: Uses comparative lasers to remove skin that is impacted.

- **Surgical Removal**: For thicker or more dubious lesions, excision or curettage is recommended.

Prospects for Further Actinic Keratosis Research

Actinic Keratosis research is still ongoing, with the goals of refining diagnostic techniques, comprehending the molecular pathways leading to SCC development, and creating less intrusive and more successful treatment options. Among the future paths are:

Finding biomarkers to determine which AKs are most likely to develop into cancer is known as **Biomarkers**.

Advanced Imaging Techniques: AK lesions can be better detected and monitored early with non-invasive imaging.

- **Immunotherapy**: Research novel immunotherapeutic drugs to strengthen the skin's defenses against aberrant cells.

Gene Therapy: Researching genetic methods to repair DNA damage caused by UV light.

Preventive Strategies: Improving sunscreens and other protective gear to avert UV damage and the consequent development of AK.

People can manage Actinic Keratosis, a common but potentially dangerous disorder, by being aware of the condition and taking proactive measures to protect their skin, recognizing early signs, and seeking timely medical attention.

CHAPTER 2

RECOGNIZING UV RADIATION AND SUN DAMAGE

A Comprehensive Guide to Actinic Keratosis: Understanding Sun Damage and UV Radiation

UV Radiation's Effects on Skin

One of the main environmental factors that impacts skin tone is ultraviolet (UV) light from the sun. UVA and UVB rays are the main forms of UV radiation that reach the surface of the Earth. These rays pierce the skin and harm the skin in several ways.

- **DNA Damage**: UV radiation can cause direct damage to skin cells' DNA, which can result in mutations that can cause actinic keratosis and other skin cancers.

- **Inflammation**: Sun exposure sets off an inflammatory reaction that results in swelling and redness (sunburn).

- **Immunological Suppression**: Prolonged exposure to UV light can inhibit the skin's local immunological response, making it less able to recognize and heal cellular damage.

- **Protein Damage**: UV rays break down proteins that are vital to the structure and suppleness of skin, such as collagen and elastin.

The Distinction Between UVA and UVB Radiation

The UVA (320–400 nm) rays:

- **Penetration**: The skin's deeper layer, up to the dermis.

Effects: Contributes to skin cancer and causes long-term skin damage such as photoaging (wrinkles, loss of suppleness).

- **Presence**: Is responsible for 95% of the UV light that reaches Earth. It may pass through glass and clouds and is generally constant in intensity throughout the day.

- **UVB Rays: 290–320 nanometers):**
- **Penetration**: Mainly impacts the epidermis, the skin's outermost layer.

- **Effects**: Causes direct DNA damage and sunburn. It contributes significantly to the development of actinic keratosis and other forms of skin cancer.

- **Presence**: Depends on location, season, and time of day. It peaks between ten in the morning. and 4 PM, particularly throughout the summer.

Photoaging and Skin Ageing

Intrinsic Ageing: The aging process that occurs naturally and is influenced by genetics.

-Photoaging: Skin aging prematurely as a result of frequent UV exposure. It is distinguished by:

Fine Lines and Wrinkles: Owing to collagen deterioration.

Age spots and freckles are examples of **hyperpigmentation**

Loss of Elasticity: Skin sagging as a result of elastin fiber degradation.

Rough Texture: The skin becomes thicker and rougher.

Actinic Keratosis and UV Exposure Relationship

A rough, scaly patch on the skin brought on by prolonged exposure to UV rays is called actinic keratosis (AK). It is regarded as precancerous because squamous cell carcinoma (SCC) could develop from it in the future. The following factors affect the development of AK:

- **Cumulative UV Exposure**: The danger rises with prolonged exposure to UV radiation.

- **Skin Type**: People with fair skin are more vulnerable.

- **Age**: Due to cumulative UV damage over time, more prevalent in older persons.

- **Immune Status**: People with compromised immune systems, such as those who have received organ transplants, are particularly vulnerable.

Sun Protection Is Crucial

To shield skin from UV rays and lower the chance of developing actinic keratosis and other skin malignancies, effective sun protection is essential. The principal causes are as follows:

- **Prevention of DNA Damage**: Lowers the possibility of cancer-causing mutations.

- **Minimising Photoaging**: Guards against wrinkles and age spots, two indicators of early aging.

- **Reducing Sunburn and Inflammation**: Prevents the painful and immediate impacts of UV radiation.

- **Preserving Immune Function**: Preserves the skin's capacity to defend against infections and heal itself.

Frequently Held Myths Regarding Sunscreen

- **SPF 50+ Means No Reapplication**: Reapplication is still necessary even with a high SPF. Reapplying sunscreen is advised every two hours, and more frequently if perspiring or swimming is involved.

- **Only Required on Sunny Days**: On cloudy days, UV radiation can still cause damage.

- **Dark Skin Doesn't Need Sunscreen**: Darker skin is still vulnerable to UV damage and skin cancer even though it has more melanin and some natural defense.

- **Sunscreen Causes Vitamin D Deficiency**: Vitamin D levels can be maintained by food and supplements; proper use of sunscreen has no discernible effect on them.

UV Index and Hazard Evaluation

The UV Index indicates the amount of UV light that might cause sunburns at a specific location and time. It aids in risk assessment and the implementation of suitable preventive measures:

- **0-2 (Low)**: Minimal risk, wear sunglasses for minimal protection.

- **3-5 (Moderate)**: Wear protective gear, seek shade during the noon hours, and there is a moderate risk.

- **6-7 (High)**: Extremely risky; limit sun exposure starting at 10 a.m. up until 4 p.m., use sunscreen.

8–10 (Very High): Very high danger; avoid the sun as much as possible and take extra precautions.

- **11+ (Extreme)**: High risk; protect yourself from the sun by using heavy sunscreen.

Strategies for Photoprotection

- **Sunscreen**: SPF 30 or higher broad-spectrum (UVA and UVB) sunscreen.

- **ATTIRE**: Don long-sleeved shirts, slacks, and hats with wide brims.

- **Sunglasses**: Use UV-blocking eyewear to protect your eyes.

Look for shade, particularly from 10 a.m. to 4 p.m. when UV exposure is at its highest.

- **Avoid Tanning Beds**: Tanning beds raise the risk of skin cancer by emitting dangerous UV radiation.

Including Sun-Safe Practices in Everyday Activities

- **Daily Sunscreen Use**: Use sunscreen daily, whether rain or shine.

- **Protective Clothes**: Whenever possible, wear apparel with a UV protection factor (UPF).

- **Regular Check-Ups**: See a dermatologist for skin exams and regularly check your skin for new or changing lesions.

- **Educate and Advocate**: Raise family and friends' knowledge of the value of sun protection.

UV Protection Public Health Initiatives

- **Education Campaigns**: Make people aware of the risks associated with UV rays and the need for protective gear.

- **School Programmes**: Encourage the use of sunscreen and protective clothing by implementing sun safety teaching in schools.

- **Policy and Regulation**: Push for laws that restrict the use of tanning beds and encourage the provision of shade in public areas.

- **Community Outreach**: Give away free sunscreen at outdoor gatherings and public events.

Research and Monitoring: Encourage studies on the relationship between UV rays and the prevention of skin cancer, and track the success of public health campaigns.

People can lessen their chance of acquiring actinic keratosis and other skin-related disorders and better protect themselves from the sun's damaging effects by being aware of these aspects of UV radiation and sun damage.

CHAPTER 3

RISK ELEMENTS AND PREVENTIVE TECHNIQUES

Of course, the following is a comprehensive guide that addresses all of the points you raised about actinic keratosis risk factors and prevention techniques:

Genetic Predisposition and Skin Type

- Fair-skinned people are more susceptible to actinic keratosis (AK) because their melanin provides less UV protection.

- Genetic factors are involved; those who have a family history of skin cancer or AK may be more vulnerable.

Causes of Actinic Keratosis in the Environment

- Extended sun exposure is important, particularly in areas with strong sunshine.

- Artificial UV radiation sources, such as tanning beds, also make a substantial contribution.

Workplace Risks and Sun Exposure

Workers outside, like farmers and construction workers, are more likely to be exposed to UV rays.

- Wearing sunscreen and wearing appropriate protection gear is essential in these types of jobs.

Living Decisions and Their Effects

Lifestyle choices like tanning beds or prolonged sun exposure increase the risk of AK.

- Poor diet and smoking can also cause damage to the skin and hinder its capacity to heal.

Immune Suppression's Role

Because immunosuppressed people, such as organ transplant recipients, have fewer immune cells to watch out for, their rates of acute rejection (AK) are higher.

Ageing and Gender Factors:

- Ageing increases the risk of AK because of cumulative sun exposure.

- Men tend to get more AK lesions than women, which may be related to disparities in sun exposure at work and during leisure time.

Prevention via Early Childhood Education

- Teaching people about sun protection from an early age can greatly lower their chance of developing AK later in life.

It is essential to teach sun protection precautions including applying sunscreen and donning protective clothes.

Behavioural Adjustments to Lower Risk:

- Promoting actions like avoiding tanning beds and looking for cover during the hottest parts of the day can help prevent AK.

Frequent skin self-examinations are crucial for identifying AK early on.

Programmes for Community-Based Prevention

- Community programs that encourage sun safety practices, supply sunscreen in public areas, and host informative workshops can lower the incidence of AK.

Prevention initiatives can be strengthened by collaborating with healthcare providers, employers, and schools.

Including Prevention In Medical Procedures:

- AK risk factors should be routinely evaluated by healthcare professionals while seeing patients.

- Promoting routine skin exams and offering advice on sun protection techniques are essential components of preventative healthcare plans.

A multifaceted strategy that targets individual behaviors, environmental variables, and community-wide actions is required to implement effective preventative strategies. Together, these factors can help lessen the effects of actinic keratosis and improve the health of your skin in general.

CHAPTER 4

CLINICAL ASSESSMENT AND IDENTIFICATION

Significance of Skin Exams

Frequent skin inspections are essential for actinic keratosis (AK) early identification and therapy. These assessments might be carried out by medical professionals or by the self. Patients who self-examine are better able to track changes in their skin, spot new lesions, and get timely medical care. Expert skin examinations, usually carried out by dermatologists, guarantee a comprehensive assessment utilizing specialized instruments and methods, resulting in precise diagnoses and suitable treatment regimens. Regular skin exams can aid in the early detection of AK and stop it from progressing to squamous cell carcinoma (SCC), a potentially aggressive form of skin cancer.

Crucial Elements for Recognising Actinic Keratosis Lesions

Actinic keratosis lesions can appear as flesh-colored, pink, or red patches and are distinguished by their rough, scaly texture. They frequently appear on sun-exposed regions of the body such as the hands, ears, neck, and scalp. Important characteristics consist of:

- **Texture**: Texturally rough, similar to sandpaper.

- **Colour**: Skin-colored, brown, pink, or red.

- **Size**: Usually tiny, with a diameter of a few millimeters to around one centimeter.

- **Shape**: May have a definite border and be flat or slightly elevated.

- **Location**: Usually found in skin regions exposed to the sun.

Although these lesions are frequently asymptomatic, they can occasionally cause itching or a prickling feeling.

Differential Diagnoses and Related Illnesses

Accurately diagnosing actinic keratosis from other skin disorders is essential for treatment planning. Conditions that exhibit comparable presentations consist of:

- **Seborrhoeic Keratosis**: Typically darker and appearing "stuck-on"

- **Squamous Cell Carcinoma (SCC)**: More invasive, bigger, and susceptible to bleeding or ulceration.

- **Basal Cell Carcinoma (BCC)**: May present with a central ulceration and a pearly appearance.

- **Psoriasis and Eczema**: Psoriasis is typically more widely distributed, while eczema is characterized by itching and silvery scales.

- **Lichenoid Keratosis**: Less likely to be scaly and usually more uniform in color.

Histopathological Examination and Biopsy Methods

To confirm the diagnosis when the clinical examination yields no clear results, a biopsy is carried out. Typical biopsy methods consist of:

- **Shave Biopsy**: Ideal for superficial lesions, this procedure removes the outermost layers of skin.

- **Punch Biopsy**: a deeper sample is taken with a circular blade to capture the entire thickness of the lesion.

- **Excisional Biopsy**: When a cancer is detected, the entire lesion is excised.

Under a microscope, the biopsy sample is examined for atypical keratinocytes restricted to the epidermis, hyperkeratosis, and parakeratosis as part of the histopathological examination. To confirm the diagnosis, further cellular abnormalities and inflammation are evaluated.

Actinic Keratosis Diagnosis Using Dermoscopy

A non-invasive imaging method called dermoscopy improves the visibility of skin lesions. Dermoscopic characteristics of actinic keratosis include:

Underlying vascular patterns in sun-damaged skin is the **Red pseudonetwork**.

- **Keratotic plugs**: Round, tiny formations inside the lesion that have a yellowish-brown color.

Strawberry pattern: A red-colored vascular pattern surrounded by white halos at the follicular apertures.

Dermoscopy enhances diagnostic precision by highlighting minute details that are invisible to the unaided eye.

Photography's Function in Tracking Injuries

Photography is a helpful tool for tracking the development or regression of actinic keratosis lesions over time, including clinical and dermoscopic photographs. Comparing lesion characteristics at various visits is made easier with the help of high-resolution photographs, which offer a visual record. This is especially helpful in identifying alterations that might point to malignant transformation. Regular photo documenting guarantees thorough and precise observation, allowing for prompt interventions.

Remote Diagnosis and Teledermatology

Utilizing technology, teledermatology offers dermatological care from a distance. It consists of:

- **Store-and-Forward**: Dermatologists get photographs and information from patients, evaluate them, and make recommendations.

- **Real-Time Consultations**: Patients and dermatologists can communicate instantly through live video consultations.

Teledermatology improves accessibility and eliminates the need for in-person visits for actinic keratosis early diagnosis and treatment, especially for patients living in distant places.

Educating Patients During the Diagnosis

Effective care of actinic keratosis requires educating patients about the condition. Important details consist of:

Risk Factors: Fair skin, history of sunburns, prolonged sun exposure, and immunosuppression.

- **Self-Examination**: How to check your skin frequently and identify AK symptoms early.

- **Sun Protection**: The significance of applying sunscreen, donning protective apparel, and steering clear of periods of high UV radiation.

Follow-Up: Consistent dermatological examinations are required to track lesions and stop them from getting worse.

Patients who receive comprehensive knowledge are more equipped to take charge of their skin health.

Diagnosis's Psychological Impact

Actinic keratosis diagnoses can have a major psychological impact, including worry about possible skin cancer progression and cosmetic concerns. Patients may feel anxious and concerned about the state of their skin, as well as the consequences of chronic sun exposure. Taking care of these psychological elements entails:

- **Counselling**: offering encouragement and confidence in the benign character of AK and practical means of therapy.

- **Communication**: To allay anxieties and set reasonable expectations, communicate straightforwardly and compassionately.

- **Support Groups**: Promoting involvement in support groups for people with comparable problems.

Using a Multidisciplinary Method to Diagnose

By combining different skills, a multidisciplinary approach improves the care of actinic keratosis:

Dermatologists: Play a major part in both diagnosis and therapy.

- **Pathologists**: Essential in analyzing biopsy samples histopathologically.

- **Oncologists**: When lesions develop into SCC.

- **Primary Care Physicians**: Consultations with dermatologists and initial screening.

- **Nurses and Physician Assistants**: Help with follow-up, minor procedures, and patient education.

Working together, healthcare professionals may guarantee patient outcomes by providing thorough care, prompt diagnosis, and efficient treatment.

CHAPTER 5

METHODS OF TREATMENT

Comprehensive Guide to Actinic Keratosis: Available Treatment Options

Actinic Keratosis Topical Treatments

The mainstay of treatment for actinic keratosis (AK) is topical therapy, particularly for those with numerous lesions or extensive afflicted areas. Usually, these therapies consist of:

1. **5-Fluorouracil (5-FU): An antimetabolite that destroys aberrant cells by interfering with DNA synthesis. It is often applied twice a day for a few weeks, during which time the skin

becomes irritated and peels, a sign that AK cells are being destroyed.

2. **Imiquimod:** Inducing the local immune system to target aberrant cells is the purpose of this immune response modulator. When used two to three times a week for a few weeks, it may result in swelling and redness on the skin in that area.

3. **Diclofenac Sodium Gel:** A cyclooxygenase enzyme-inhibiting nonsteroidal anti-inflammatory medication (NSAID) that decreases cell division. When contrast to 5-FU, it often causes milder adverse effects and is given twice daily for 60–90 days.

4. **Ingenol Mebutate:** Derived from the Euphorbia peplus plant's sap, it triggers an

immunological reaction and cell death. Although the treatment course is brief—applying for two to three days on average—it can have a considerable local reaction.

Because they are non-invasive, topical treatments are popular for treating apparent and subclinical lesions in the field.

Techniques for Cryotherapy and Cryosurgery

Liquid nitrogen is applied during cryotherapy to freeze and kill aberrant cells. This method is frequently applied to differentiate AK lesions.

1. **Procedure:** Applying liquid nitrogen with a cotton-tipped applicator or spray device causes the lesion and surrounding skin to quickly freeze. The size and thickness of the

lesion determine how long the therapy takes, which can be anything from a few seconds to more than a minute.

2. **Efficacy and Side Effects:** With a success rate of up to 99%, cryotherapy is incredibly successful in treating single lesions. Blisters, discomfort, and possible hypopigmentation or scarring at the treatment site are examples of side effects.

Cryosurgery is a first-line treatment for isolated lesions due to its benefits, including rapidity, effectiveness, and little aftercare.

Photodynamic Therapy (PDT)

Using a photosensitizing drug in conjunction with light exposure, photodynamic treatment targets and kills aberrant cells.

1. **Procedure:** The affected area is covered with a topical photosensitizer, such as methyl aminolevulinate (MAL) or aminolevulinic acid (ALA), and left to incubate for one to three hours. After that, the region is subjected to a particular wavelength of light, which causes the photosensitizer to become active and release reactive oxygen species, which kill AK cells.

2. **Efficacy and Side Effects:** With a clearance rate of roughly 70–90%, PDT is useful for treating individual lesions as well as fields. Erythema, peeling after therapy, and discomfort during light exposure are among the side effects.

PDT is prized for its capacity to treat both overt and covert lesions, and for producing often more favorable cosmetic results than alternative methods.

Options for Laser Treatment

Lasers can destroy AK lesions precisely and deliberately while causing the least amount of tissue damage possible.

1. **Lighting Types:**

- **Carbon Dioxide (CO2) Laser:** Minimises bleeding and vaporises the lesion. Although it involves local anesthesia and can cause substantial agony, it is incredibly effective.

- **Erbium: YAG Laser:** Promotes faster healing through controlled ablation with reduced thermal damage compared to CO2 lasers.

2. **Efficacy and Side Effects:** Although laser treatments have a high clearance rate, there is a chance of scarring, edema, and erythema following the procedure.

Patients seeking precise, cosmetically pleasing results and those with larger or resistant lesions can benefit most from laser treatment.

Surgical Removal and Resection

AK lesions that are thicker, more suspicious, or recurrent are only treated surgically.

1. **Excision:** Usually done under local anesthesia, the lesion and a margin of surrounding tissue are surgically removed. With the help of this technique, tissue can be

examined histopathologically to rule out invasive cancer.

2. **Curettage:** Uses a curette to scrape the lesion; electrosurgery is frequently used to kill any remaining aberrant cells. Although this method is rapid and efficient, scarring could occur.

Surgical techniques are quite successful, although they are usually employed in cases where no other treatment works or where cancer is suspected.

Chemical Peels for the Treatment of Actinic Keratosis

To encourage the regeneration of healthy skin, chemical peels entail applying a chemical solution to the epidermis and a portion of the dermis.

1. Peel Types:

- **Superficial Peels:** To remove the outermost layer of skin, use alpha hydroxy acids (AHAs) or beta hydroxy acids (BHAs).

- **Medium Peels:** To reach the mid-dermis, apply trichloroacetic acid (TCA).

- **Deep Peels:** To induce greater tissue breakdown and deeper penetration, use phenol.

2. **Efficacy and Side Effects:** Chemical peels work well for treating many AKs and enhancing the texture of the skin generally. Redness, peeling, and possible hyperpigmentation or scarring are examples of side effects.

Chemical peels are a good option for treating large areas of sun-damaged skin while treating field cancer.

Agents Immunomodulatory

These substances improve the immune system's capacity to identify and eliminate aberrant cells.

1. **Models:**

- **Imiquimod:** When applied topically, it stimulates Toll-like receptor 7, which results in the production of cytokines and the infiltration of immune cells.

- **Interferon:** Injecting interferon directly into lesions might sometimes boost the immune response locally.

2. **Efficacy and Side Effects:** Immunomodulatory drugs can remove AK lesions efficiently, but they may also have serious local skin reactions, such as swelling, redness, and flu-like symptoms.

When other therapies are prohibited or a patient has many lesions, these medicines are especially helpful.

Combination Treatments for Immune Toxins

Several therapy techniques together can improve results, particularly for AK lesions that are resistant.

1. **Models:**

- **Cryotherapy with Topical 5-FU:** This combination of topical chemotherapy and mechanical destruction improves overall clearance rates.

- **PDT with Imiquimod:** By combining photodynamic activity with immune modulation, sequential administration enhances both short- and long-term results.

2. **Efficacy and Side Effects:** Combination treatments frequently result in greater clearance

rates, but they also carry a larger risk of negative side effects, necessitating cautious patient selection and close observation.

Combination techniques maximize therapy results by being customized to each patient's needs.

Algorithms and Guidelines for Treatment

Clinical guidelines provide evidence-based and standardized care by providing a framework for the management of AK.

1. **Thoughts:**

- **Lesion Characteristics:** AK lesions' size, thickness, quantity, and placement.

Patient preferences, age, immunological condition, and comorbidities are examples of patient factors.

2. **Guidelines:** For resistant or suspicious lesions, generally suggest beginning with the least invasive choices (e.g., topical treatments, cryotherapy) and working your way up to more invasive techniques (e.g., PDT, laser, surgery).

Following treatment guidelines guarantees methodical and efficient care of AK.

Post-treatment patient monitoring and follow-up

For early diagnosis of recurrence or advancement to squamous cell carcinoma, routine follow-up is essential.

1. **Timetable:**

- **First Follow-Up:** Usually conducted 4-6 weeks following therapy to evaluate effectiveness and adverse effects.

- **Long-Term Monitoring:** based on treatment response and individual risk factors, every 6–12 months.

2. **Assessment:** Consists of a comprehensive skin examination as well as patient education regarding sun protection and self-monitoring.

The management of long-term hazards associated with AK and the prevention of recurrence depends heavily on ongoing monitoring and patient education.

Healthcare professionals can effectively manage actinic keratosis, increasing patient outcomes and lowering the risk of skin cancer progression, by being aware of and utilizing these diverse treatment options.

CHAPTER 6

HANDLING ACTINIC KERATOSIS IN PARTICULAR GROUPS

Pediatric Patients with Actinic Keratosis:

Compared to adults, pediatric patients had a lower incidence of actinic keratosis, primarily as a result of less sun exposure and shorter cumulative UV exposure. When it develops, though, it frequently causes concern since it may lead to the development of skin cancer in the future. To lower the risk of development, management entails teaching carers about sun protection, conducting routine skin exams, and treating lesions as soon as possible.

Geriatric Issues and Difficulties:

Actinic keratosis in elderly adults frequently manifests as many comorbidities, and they may be on multiple drugs. To ensure efficacy and minimize side effects, treatment decisions must take these considerations into account. As older people may have compromised skin barrier function and decreased capacity to tolerate certain therapies, routine follow-ups and monitoring are essential.

In Immunocompromised Individuals: Actinic Keratosis

People with impaired immune systems, such as those receiving organ transplants or living with HIV/AIDS, are more vulnerable to actinic keratosis and the skin malignancies that can follow. To detect and treat lesions promptly, management entails a multidisciplinary strategy that includes close monitoring, customized treatment programs, and routine dermatologic exams.

Managing Actinic Keratosis During Pregnancy:

Pregnancy-related actinic keratosis management needs to be carefully considered because there are possible dangers involved with some treatment options. Topical treatments like imiquimod may be taken into consideration under strict medical care during pregnancy, while choices like cryotherapy and 5-fluorouracil are typically avoided.

Differences in Presentation by Culture and Ethnicity:

Actinic keratosis appearance and perception might be affected by cultural and ethnic differences. There can be significant differences in skin type, UV sensitivity, and attitudes towards skin health amongst various populations. Effective prevention and management techniques require addressing cultural attitudes and practices through the customization of outreach and education programs.

Access to Care and Socioeconomic Factors:

People with actinic keratosis may find it difficult to receive the care they need due to socioeconomic considerations. Delays in diagnosis and treatment might be caused by a lack of health insurance, economic hurdles, and restricted access to dermatological treatments. Collaboration between community organizations, legislators, and healthcare providers is necessary to remove these obstacles.

Patient Psychological Support:

Patients may experience worry and emotional discomfort as a result of their actinic keratosis diagnosis and treatment. Offering psychological support can enhance a patient's quality of life and results. This help can include information on the ailment, coping mechanisms, and connections to support groups.

Approaches in Integrated Medicine:

Actinic keratosis treatments may be complemented by integrative medicine strategies like dietary changes, stress-reduction methods, and complementary therapies like acupuncture. However there isn't much data to support their effectiveness in treating this particular ailment, so they should only be taken as a supplement to conventional medical care.

Advanced Cases: Palliative Care

Palliative care is for patients with advanced actinic keratosis who have considerable symptoms or who are at risk of developing skin cancer. Its goals include managing symptoms, enhancing quality of life, and supporting patients and their families emotionally. This could involve end-of-life planning, wound care, and pain management.

Family and Carer Support:

Patients with actinic keratosis may also affect their family members and carers. Providing carers with information, tools, and support promotes treatment plan adherence, continuity of care, and general patient and support network well-being.

CHAPTER 7

ISSUES AND PROLONGED CONSEQUENCES

A Comprehensive Guide on Actinic Keratosis: Long-Term Consequences and Complications

A common skin ailment called actinic keratosis (AK) is brought on by extended exposure to ultraviolet (UV) radiation, usually from the sun. It can develop into more severe conditions and appears as rough, scaly patches on skin exposed to the sun. For efficient management and patient care, it is essential to comprehend the long-term consequences and problems of AK.

Squamous Cell Carcinoma Progression

It is thought that actinic keratosis precedes squamous cell carcinoma (SCC). If treatment is not received, 10–15% of AK lesions may develop into SCC. The significance of early detection and intervention is emphasized by this development. Timely treatment of AK is crucial to prevent the malignant transition into SCC, a more invasive form of skin cancer that has the potential to spread to deeper tissues and other parts of the body.

Advanced Lesions' Metastatic Potential

Most AK lesions are benign, but those that progress to SCC have the potential to become invasive. Advanced SCC can spread to distant organs and lymph nodes. Because metastatic

SCC is linked to increased rates of morbidity and mortality, it requires rigorous therapy and vigilant monitoring. The chance of acquiring metastatic SCC can be greatly decreased by treating AK early and well.

Rates of Recurrence Following Treatment

Following therapy, AK recurrence is frequent; the rate of recurrence varies based on the technique used. One of the most popular therapies, cryotherapy, has a recurrence rate of 5–10%. There are differences in the recurrence rates of other treatments, including photodynamic therapy, laser treatments, and topical medicines (such as imiquimod and 5-fluorouracil). To effectively manage recurrent lesions, maintenance treatments, and ongoing surveillance are frequently necessary.

Cosmetic Concerns and Scar Formation

Scarring may occur from AK treatments, particularly those involving cryotherapy or surgical excision. For many patients, the cosmetic result is a major concern, especially if the lesions are on places that are visible, such as the hands or face. To reduce scarring, advanced therapeutic methods and good wound care are recommended. It is important to advise patients on various scar treatment strategies as well as possible cosmetic outcomes.

Functional Deficit Owing to Injuries

When AK lesions develop on the lips (actinic cheilitis) or eyelids, for example, they may lead to functional impairment. Damage in these areas might make it difficult to carry out daily tasks like speaking, eating, and seeing. It might be necessary to remove these lesions surgically and to restore appearance and functionality, reconstructive surgeries might be needed.

Effect of Psychology on Life Quality

The requirement for continuous treatment due to the chronic nature of AK can have a substantial psychological effect on individuals. Anxiety and a lower quality of life might result from worries about the spread of cancer, one's physical appearance, and the necessity of frequent medical appointments. Some of these worries can be reduced by offering comfort, information, and psychological support. Counseling services and support groups could also be helpful.

Monitoring Techniques for Patients at High Risk

Patients are more likely to develop new lesions and SCC if they have a history of AK, significant UV damage, or skin cancer. Dermatological examinations regularly, often every three to six months, are advised for these high-risk patients. In-depth skin exams are performed during these appointments to identify any new or recurring lesions as soon as possible. To keep an eye on questionable areas, dermatoscopy and, in certain situations, biopsy may be used.

Supplementary Preventive Actions

Reducing the likelihood of recurrence and the formation of new AK lesions is the main goal of secondary prevention strategies. Among these actions are:

- **Sun Protection**: Avoiding peak sun exposure, wearing protective clothes, and using broad-spectrum sunscreens consistently.

- **Topical Treatments**: Applying topical medications, such as retinoids, might lessen the development of new lesions.

- **Patient Education**: teaching patients how to examine their skin and stressing the value of routine dermatological exams.

Long-Term Results Research

Research on the efficacy of different treatment methods and their effects on quality of life is being conducted to gain a better understanding of the long-term results of patients with AK. Targeted therapeutics may be developed as a result of research into the genetic and molecular pathways underpinning the progression from

AK to SCC. The best ways to stop progression and recurrence must be identified through long-term follow-up research.

Attending to Patient Worries Regarding Complications

To address patient concerns regarding problems associated with AK, effective communication is essential. The advantages, disadvantages, and possible side effects of different treatments should be explained in clear, comprehensive terms by healthcare professionals. Giving patients access to trustworthy internet resources, writing materials, and visual aids can help them comprehend their disease and available treatments. In addition to reducing patient fear, encouraging questions and dialogue during consultations helps promote a team-based approach to patient treatment.

In summary, treating actinic keratosis requires a thorough strategy that takes into account the condition's possible side effects and long-term consequences. Healthcare professionals can greatly enhance the prognosis of patients with AK via early discovery, efficient treatment, ongoing monitoring, and patient education.

CHAPTER 8

Instruction for Patients and Self-Management

Comprehensive Handbook on Actinic Keratosis

Patient Education Is Critical for Actinic Keratosis

To effectively manage actinic keratosis (AK), patients must be empowered to comprehend their illness, identify symptoms early, and participate actively in their treatment regimen. Patients with greater knowledge are more likely to follow treatment plans and preventive measures, which lowers the chance that AK may develop into SCC. By eradicating misconceptions and lowering fear, knowledge about AK also empowers patients to make wise decisions regarding their care.

Comprehending the Objectives and Treatment Options

Treatments for actinic keratosis are intended to get rid of lesions, stop them from coming back, and lower the chance that they will turn into skin cancer. Options for treatment consist of:

- **Topical Medications**: These aid in the destruction of aberrant cells and include imiquimod, diclofenac, and 5-fluorouracil (5-FU).

- **Cryotherapy**: This procedure uses liquid nitrogen to freeze the lesions, causing them to fall off.

- **Photodynamic Therapy (PDT)**: The skin is treated with a photosensitizing substance, which is then light-activated to kill aberrant cells.

- **Chemical Peels**: Targeting AK lesions, acidic solutions are used to remove the skin's outer layers.

- **Laser Therapy**: The afflicted skin layers are evaporated using ablative lasers.

Removing visible lesions, reducing side effects, and preserving skin health are the objectives.

Methods for Self-Examination

Self-examinations regularly are crucial for spotting new or evolving lesions early on. Patients ought to:

1. **Examine All Skin regions**: Check every part of the body, including regions that are difficult to view, such as the back, scalp, and soles of the feet, using a mirror.

2. **Look for Changes**: Make a note of any previously existing places that have changed or any new, rough, scaly patches.

3. **Photographic Records**: To monitor changes over time, periodically snap pictures of questionable regions.

4. **Regular Frequency**: Conduct monthly self-examinations.

Sun Safety Procedures for Everyday Living

Sun protection is essential for AK prevention. Among the efficient methods are:

Apply sunscreen with a minimum SPF of 30 and reapply it every two hours, or after swimming or perspiring.

Protective Apparel: Put on UV-blocking sunglasses, wide-brimmed hats, and long sleeves.

- **Shadow**: Look for shade from 10 a.m. and 4:00 p.m. during the peak of the sun's rays.

- **Avoid Tanning Beds**: The UV rays emitted by these beds can raise your risk of developing AK.

Changes in Lifestyle to Prevent

Making the following lifestyle adjustments can dramatically lower your risk of having AK:

- **Diet**: Eat a diet high in fruits, vegetables, and omega-3 fatty acids, as well as other antioxidant-rich foods.

- **Hydration**: To keep your skin hydrated and healthy, drink lots of water.

Regular Visits with the Dermatologist: Make an appointment for an annual examination, particularly if you have a history of skin cancer or prolonged sun exposure.

- **Avoid Smoking**: Smoking raises the risk of skin lesions and can hinder skin healing.

Tracking and Reporting Modifications to Lesions

Patients should keep a close eye on any changes to current skin lesions or the emergence of new ones. Report the following to a healthcare provider as soon as possible:

- **Size Changes**: A lesion that enlarges or elevates.

Colour Changes: A shift in hue or darkening of color.

- **Texture Changes**: The skin may become thicker, crustier, or scaled.

Symptoms: Tenderness, itching, or bleeding.

Following Treatment Plans

For AK to be managed effectively, medication regimen adherence is crucial. Among the techniques to improve adherence are:

- **Understanding the Regimen**: Make sure you have clear directions on how to take prescription drugs or adhere to treatment plans.

- **Managing Side Effects**: Talk to a healthcare professional about possible side effects and strategies to lessen them.

- **Support Systems**: Enlist the help of carers or family members to promote adherence.

Patient Support Resources

Making use of the resources at hand can yield more information and assistance:

- **Support Groups**: Participate in local or online support groups for people with skin cancer or AK.

- **Learning Resources**: Visit websites, videos, and pamphlets from reliable sources, such as the American Academy of Dermatology.

- **Professional Organisations**: For more resources and information, get in touch with groups like the Skin Cancer Foundation.

Providing Knowledge To Empower Patients

Well-informed patients can take charge of their health. A proactive approach is fostered by educating patients on the nature of AK, its causes, therapies, and preventive measures. Better health outcomes and greater confidence in controlling the condition are the results of this empowerment.

Formulating Customised Treatment Programmes

The treatment plan for each patient should be customized to meet their unique needs, accounting for:

- **Medical History**: Take into account prior medical interventions, treatment outcomes, and general health.

- **Lifestyle Factors**: Evaluate your everyday activities, occupation, and sun exposure.

- **Preferences and Concerns**: Take into account the wishes of the patient and attend to any worries they might have.

Regular Follow-Up: Make follow-up appointments to assess the patient's progress and make any required adjustments to the care plan.

A thorough, customized strategy guarantees that every patient gets the best possible care that fits their needs.

CHAPTER NINE

POLICY ASPECTS OF PUBLIC HEALTH

Actinic Keratosis's Cost to Healthcare Systems

Globally, actinic keratosis (AK) poses a substantial burden to healthcare systems. AK is a common skin disorder that is mainly caused by prolonged ultraviolet (UV) radiation and is characterized by rough, scaly patches on sun-exposed parts of the skin. Early detection and treatment are essential since this condition is thought to be a precursor to squamous cell carcinoma (SCC), a kind of skin cancer that is not melanoma.

Incidence and Prevalence:

In areas with significant UV exposure, the prevalence of AK rises with age, impacting up to 60% of people over 60. The incidence of AK is rising due to an aging population and more outdoor activities, especially in nations with higher UV index levels.

Medical Service Usage:

Dermatologists frequently see patients with AK on several occasions for diagnosis, follow-up, and treatment. Physical tests, biopsies, topical treatments, cryotherapy, and photodynamic therapy are all included in this. In public healthcare systems especially, these recurrent medical visits put pressure on dermatology services and lengthen appointment wait times.

Medical Expenses:

Significant expenses are associated with managing AK, including indirect (time away from work, transportation) and direct medical costs (consultations, treatments, drugs). The annual direct costs of treating AK patients reach $1 billion in the United States alone. The requirement for ongoing monitoring and care adds to the long-term budgetary strain on healthcare systems.

Actinic Keratosis's Economic Impact

Out-of-pocket expenses:

The medical expenditures associated with AK diagnosis and treatment are included in the direct costs. These consist of consultations with dermatologists, biopsies for diagnostic purposes, and various treatments including cryotherapy, topical chemotherapy drugs (such as 5-fluorouracil), and photodynamic therapy. These treatments can have a significant combined effect, particularly for patients who have many lesions.

Adverse Expenses:

Indirect costs are linked to lost productivity as a result of time missed from work for doctor's appointments and recuperation following medical procedures. There are additional expenses for providing care and for transportation. A lower quality of life may result from the psychological effects of AK and its possible progression to SCC, which would further reduce economic output.

Economic Burden Over Time:

The expenses increase if AK develops into SCC because more extensive care, possible hospital stays, and difficult surgeries become necessary. Thus, these long-term economic effects can be lessened by early and efficient management of AK.

Health Policies to Prevent Skin Cancer

Avoidance Techniques:

Skin cancer prevention health policies place a strong emphasis on educating the public about the dangers of UV radiation and the value of taking precautions such as applying sunscreen, donning protective clothes, and staying away from tanning salons. Additionally essential are early detection initiatives and routine skin examinations.

Legal Framework and Regulations:

Governments have the authority to impose laws restricting the use of tanning beds, particularly by children, and to enforce outdoor workers' occupational safety requirements. Reducing UV exposure can also be achieved by policies that support urban planning that improves shaded areas in public areas.

Health Promotion Initiatives:

Public health programs can arrange frequent skin cancer screening activities and offer free or subsidized sunscreen, particularly in high-risk communities. Incorporating instruction on skin health into school curricula helps establish lifetime protective behaviors at a young age.

The Function of NGOs and the Government in Awareness Campaigns

Programmes of the Government:

Governments can start national initiatives to raise awareness of the dangers of UV radiation and the value of early identification of AK and other skin cancers. Public service announcements, social media, radio, and television are just a few of the media platforms that these campaigns may use.

Donations from NGOs:**

The role of non-governmental organizations (NGOs) in enhancing government initiatives is crucial. They can set up outreach programs for the community, give out instructional materials, and offer screening services for free or at a reduced cost. NGOs aim to reach and impact a wider audience by concentrating on underprivileged and high-risk populations.

Partnership Initiatives:

Governments, non-governmental organizations, and healthcare providers working together can increase the impact of awareness initiatives. Collaborative efforts can combine resources, exchange knowledge, and guarantee unified messaging, resulting in increased public involvement and modifications in behavior.

Availability of Screening and Treatment Facilities

Access Obstacles:

Access to screening and treatment for AK is hampered by several factors, including lack of knowledge, socioeconomic inequality, geographic restrictions—particularly in rural areas—and a shortage of dermatology specialists. These obstacles may make it more likely that SCC may develop as a result of delayed identification and treatment.

Enhancing Usability:

Teledermatology can improve dermatological treatment accessibility by enabling early AK diagnosis and remote consultations. Underprivileged areas might receive screening and treatment services from outreach initiatives and mobile clinics. Financial barriers can be reduced by offering treatments through public healthcare systems and with subsidies.

Education and Materials:

Increasing early diagnosis rates can be achieved by teaching primary care physicians how to identify and treat AK. It's also crucial to guarantee that healthcare facilities have the infrastructure and resources needed to properly manage AK.

Insurance Protection for the Management of Actinic Keratosis

Difference in Coverage:

AK management insurance coverage varies greatly depending on the nation and insurance company. While many medical treatments are covered by some health insurance policies, others might only cover a portion of the total cost or require patients to pay a large amount out of pocket.

Recommendations for Policy:

Enacting laws supporting full insurance coverage for AK management can guarantee that patients receive the right care at the right time. To reduce patients' financial difficulties, this covers a variety of treatment alternatives, diagnostic tests, and routine screenings.

Legislation and Advocacy:

Legislative reforms to require insurance coverage for AK management may be pursued through advocacy campaigns. Decisions about policy and insurance practices can also be influenced by public knowledge of the significance of insurance coverage for skin disorders.

Priorities and Funding for Research

Needs for Research:

Funding for research is essential for comprehending the pathophysiology of AK, creating less intrusive and more effective treatments, and advancing early detection techniques. Priorities include investigating preventive measures, streamlining treatment regimens, and researching genetic and environmental risk factors.

Sources of Funding:

Government health departments, research councils, nonprofits, and investments from the private sector are some sources of funding. Collaborative research projects can benefit from the resources and knowledge of many stakeholders.

Research in Translation:

A focus on translational research can guarantee the prompt and efficient application of scientific discoveries in clinical settings. To enhance patient outcomes, funding should be provided for implementation studies and clinical trials in addition to basic research.

Promoting the Avoidance of Skin Cancer

Increasing Conscience:

Through educational initiatives, neighborhood gatherings, and collaborations with businesses and educational institutions, advocacy groups can increase public awareness of the significance of skin cancer prevention. Showcasing the individual accounts of skin cancer survivors may potentially strike a chord with the general audience.

Advocacy for Policy:

Campaigns have the power to persuade decision-makers to give skin cancer prevention a priority on public health agendas. This includes advocating for laws that encourage preventative care, providing funds for studies and screening initiatives, and ensuring that preventive care is covered by insurance.

Involvement in Community:

Involving local populations in preventative initiatives can promote a culture of skin health consciousness. It is possible to organize community leaders and influencers to disseminate information and promote preventive behaviors.

CHAPTER 10

UPCOMING DEVELOPMENTS AND TRENDS

Of course! This is a comprehensive guide to upcoming developments and advances in actinic keratosis (AK), with an emphasis on the issues listed below.

Technological Developments in Actinic Keratosis Detection

**1. Imaging Methodologies: **

Confocal Laser Scanning Microscopy (CLSM): This non-invasive imaging method offers high-resolution images that aid in the distinction between benign and malignant skin lesions. It enables the in vivo analysis of skin lesions at a cellular level.

- **Optical Coherence Tomography (OCT):** OCT assists in the early detection and monitoring of AK by using light waves to create three-dimensional, micrometer-resolution pictures from within optical scattering media, including the skin.

2. Molecular Pathology:

Biomarker Development: The identification of certain biomarkers linked to AK can improve early detection and forecast the development of SCC. Methods such as liquid biopsy, which examines tumor DNA in circulation, may prove to be essential.

3. Integration of Artificial Intelligence (AI):

- **AI Algorithms:** By analyzing huge databases of skin image data, AI and machine learning algorithms can increase the consistency and accuracy of diagnoses. Artificial intelligence (AI) systems can recognize minute details in photos that human eyes might overlook, assisting in early identification and treatment choices.

Personalised medicine and targeted therapies

1. **Genetic Profiling

- **Personalised Treatment Plans:** Treatments can be customized to target particular mutations and pathways involved in AK, improving efficacy and minimizing side effects, by knowing the genetic composition of a patient's skin lesions.

2. Medicinal Route Inhibitors:

Signal Transduction Inhibitors: More potent treatments may be obtained by focusing on particular pathways, such as the Hedgehog signaling pathway, which is connected to the onset of AK.

Development of Vaccines and Immunotherapy

1. Agents that Modulate Immunity:

- **Topical Immunotherapy:** For maximum efficacy, agents such as imiquimod, which elicit the body's immune response to attack and eliminate aberrant cells, are being honed and mixed with other therapies.

**2. Immunisations: **

Prophylactic Vaccines: Vaccines that target human papillomavirus (HPV) and other contributory factors are being developed to prevent the formation of AKs in the first place.

- **Therapeutic Vaccines:** Vaccines are meant to increase immunity to identify and eliminate pre-existing AK cells.

Treatment Applications of Nanotechnology

**1. Nanocarriers: **

Targeted Drug Delivery: Therapeutic medicines can be delivered to the lesion site directly using nanoparticles, thereby reducing systemic side effects and optimizing local efficacy.

- **Controlled Release:** Drugs can be released from nanocarriers gradually over time, increasing treatment compliance and results.

2. Improvement of Photodynamic Therapy (PDT):

- **Nano-photosensitizers:** By enhancing the delivery and activation of photosensitizing chemicals utilized in PDT, nanotechnology can shorten treatment durations and increase treatment efficacy.

Dermatology and Artificial Intelligence

**1. Tools for Diagnosis: **

Deep Learning algorithms: State-of-the-art AI algorithms are capable of reliably identifying AKs and differentiating them from other skin disorders by analyzing dermoscopic images.

- **Predictive Analytics:** AI can assist in predicting the chance that AK will proceed to SCC, directing treatment choices and aftercare plans.

**2. Planning for Treatment: **

- **AI-Driven Recommendations:** Based on patient history, lesion characteristics, and therapy response, AI systems can help dermatologists choose the best course of action.

Digital health and telemedicine solutions

1. Online Consultations:

- **Teledermatology:** By enabling virtual consultations, patients can obtain professional assessments and treatment regimens, improving access to care, particularly in underprivileged areas.

- **Mobile Apps:** Apps that let users keep track of their skin lesions, get treatment reminders, and see how they progress over time.

2. Digital Surveillance:

- **Wearable Devices:** Wearables that track UV exposure and skin changes can give patients and medical professionals access to real-time data, which can help manage lesions that already exist and stop AK from developing.

Comprehensive Methods for Skin Health

**1. Living Style and Preventive Steps:

Nutrition and Supplements: Studies on the effects of food and certain nutrients on the prevention of AK and skin health.

- **UV Protection Strategies:** Advancements in sunscreen and UV-blocking apparel that provide superior defense against UV rays.

**2. Comprehensive Care:

- **Integrative Therapies:** Improving overall skin health and patient well-being by combining traditional treatments with complementary therapies including acupuncture, herbal medicines, and stress management approaches.

Innovations Focused on the Patient

1. Instruction and Assistance:

- **Patient Portals:** Digital platforms provide access to private medical records, support groups, and educational materials.

- **Interactive Tools:** Resources that enhance patient adherence and results by educating patients about their condition and available treatments.

2. Tailored Care Programmes:

Patient Engagement: Including patients in the decision-making process to guarantee that their lifestyle and preferences are met by the treatments they get.

Ethical Aspects in Practice and Research

1. **Informed Consent

Transparency: Making certain that medical professionals are fully aware of the advantages and disadvantages of novel tools and therapies.

- **Data Privacy:** Protecting patient information, particularly when utilizing telemedicine and AI technologies.

**2. Parity in Availability:

Addressing Disparities: Making sure that all populations, including those in low-resource settings, have access to advancements in detection and treatment.

Redefining Actinic Keratosis Treatment in the Future

1. Joint Research:

- **Multi-Disciplinary Approaches:** Cooperation to improve knowledge and care for AK among dermatologists, oncologists, geneticists, and researchers.

- **Global Initiatives:** International collaborations to address AK as a worldwide health concern, encouraging treatment equity and preventive actions.

**2. Advocacy and Policy: **

- **Regulatory Frameworks:** Creating guidelines to encourage the use of cutting-edge technologies while maintaining patient security.

Public Health Campaigns: Educating the public on the significance of receiving treatment, early detection, and prevention of AK.

In conclusion, the combination of state-of-the-art technology, personalized medicine, and patient-centered approaches holds great promise for the future of actinic keratosis treatment. Ethics and fair access continue to be at the forefront of these advancements, which promise to enhance diagnosis, treatment outcomes, and general skin health.

Made in the USA
Columbia, SC
23 April 2025